Published by White Feather Press. (www.whitefeatherpress.com)

ISBN 978-1618081599

Printed in the United States of America

White Feather Press

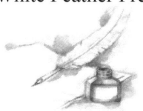

Reaffirming Faith in God, Family and Country

A note from the author

I grew up in an environment where guns were seen only in movies and TV, and the only people allowed to actually use a gun were police officers. The thought of an individual citizen actually owning a firearm for protection never occurred to me until I got married. People would constantly ask me after I purchased my first gun, "How can you buy a gun? You have two children in the house! Aren't you afraid of accidents?" Those questions were answered with two simple questions of my own.

"Where do you suggest I teach my children about gun culture in America? Should I leave that to the media and Hollywood?"

There was no response.

This book is meant not as an in-depth breakdown of guns or living with guns, but as an introduction to the world of firearms for children. Its goal is to plant the seeds of safe gun ownership into the minds of young patriots who will one day be responsible gun owners like the parents who teach them. It is up to the moms and dads of this country who exercise their 2nd Amendment rights to instill a deep respect for firearms. This book serves as the tool to open a dialogue between you and your child about keeping their "Safety On."

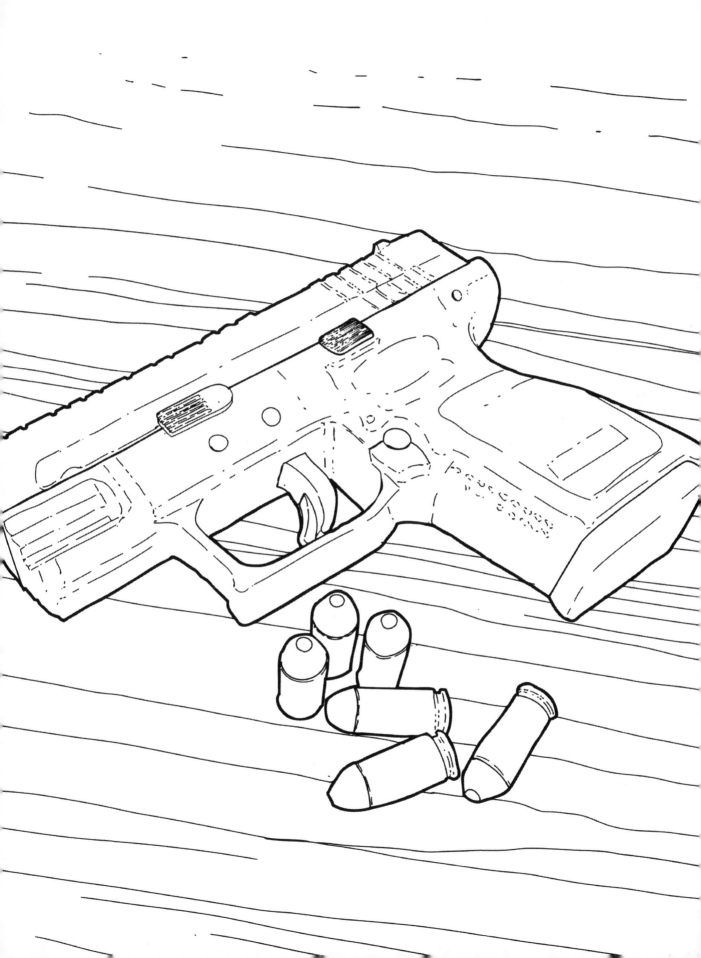

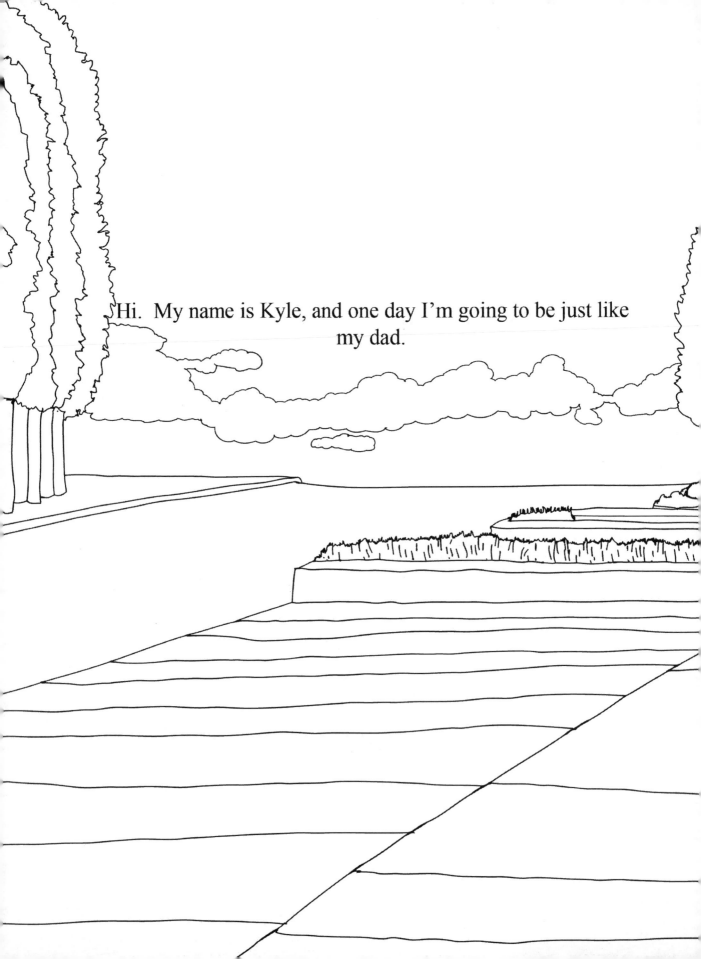

Hi. My name is Kyle, and one day I'm going to be just like my dad.

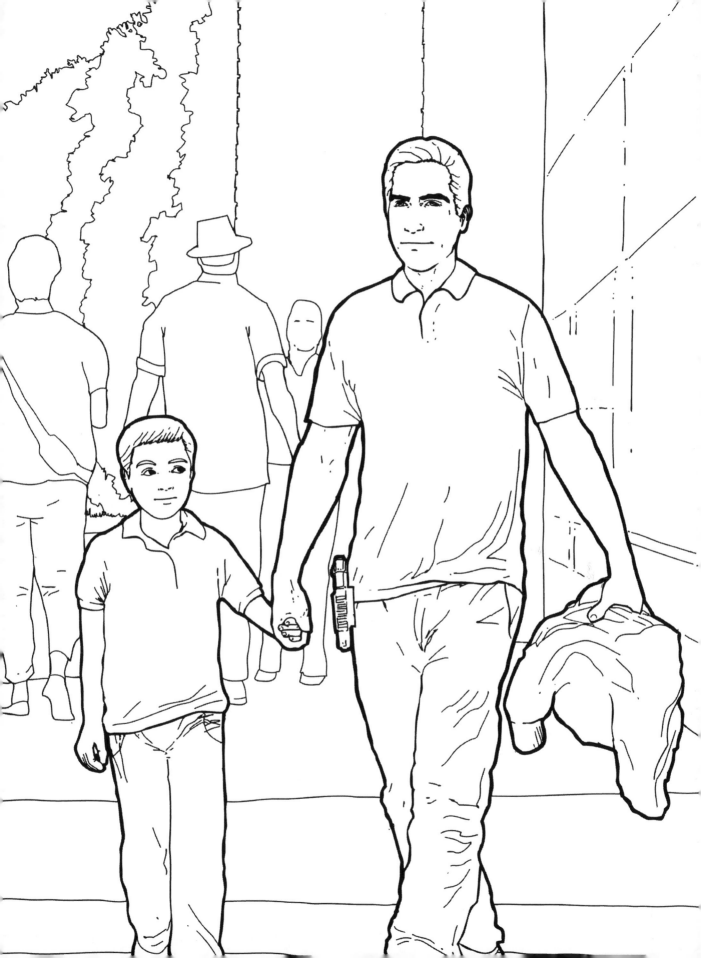

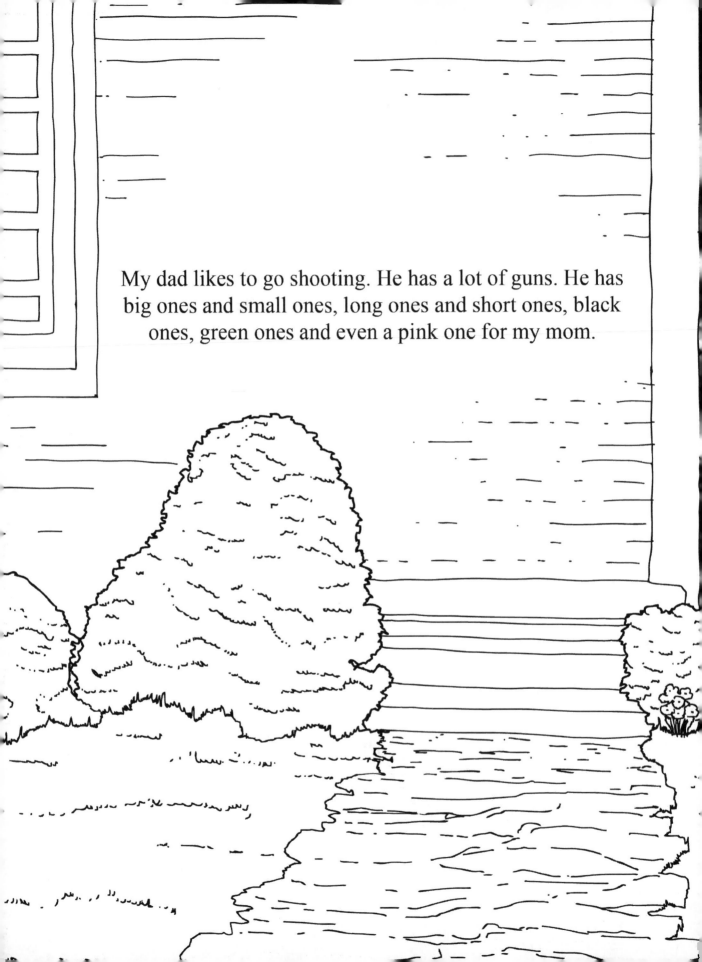

My dad likes to go shooting. He has a lot of guns. He has big ones and small ones, long ones and short ones, black ones, green ones and even a pink one for my mom.

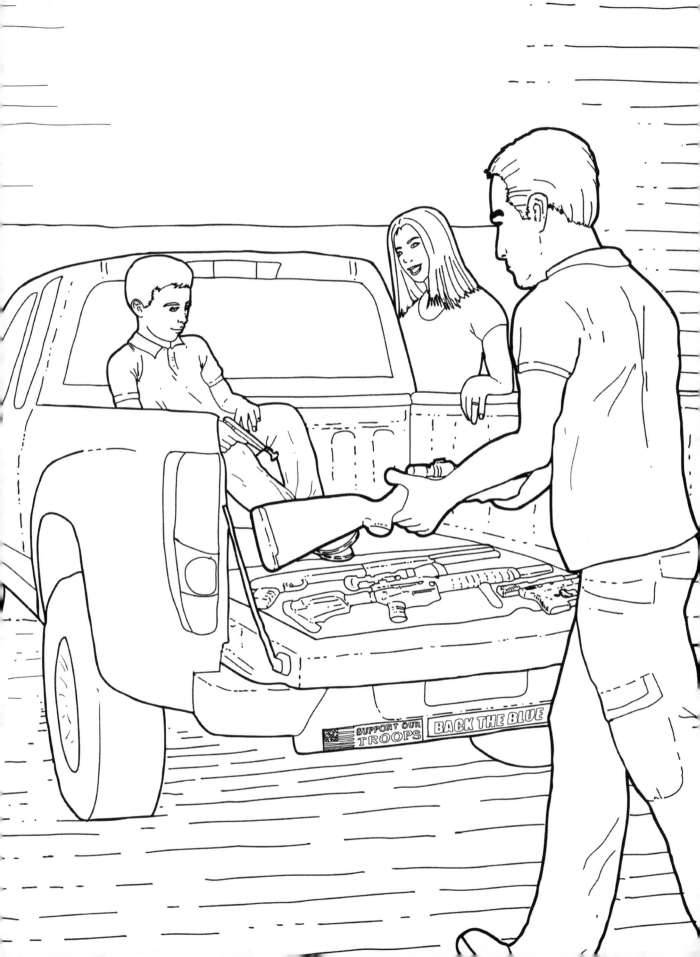

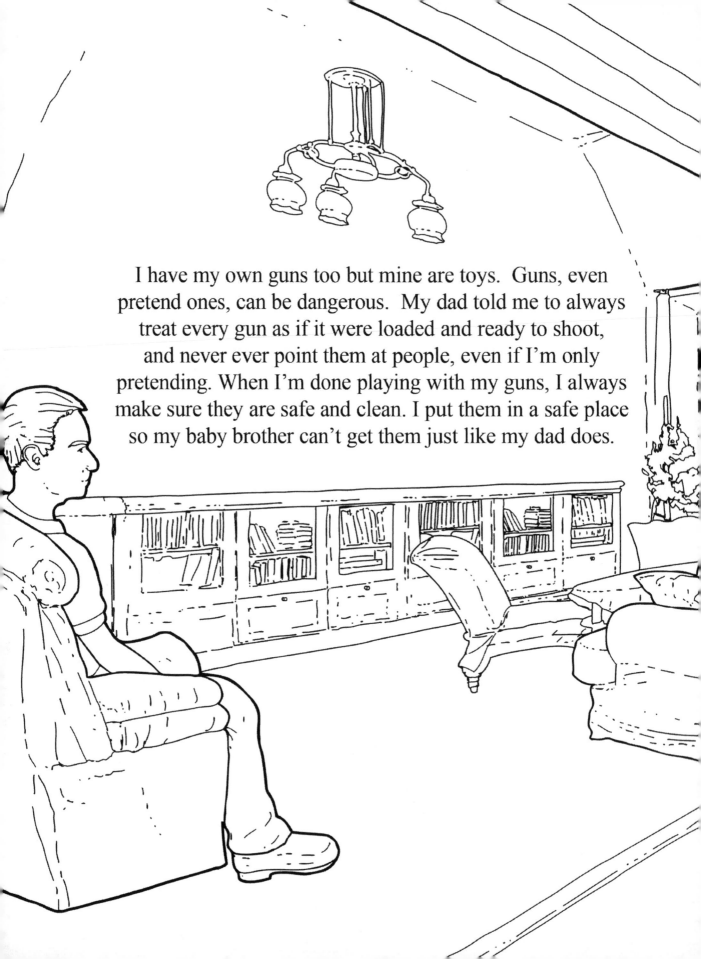

I have my own guns too but mine are toys. Guns, even pretend ones, can be dangerous. My dad told me to always treat every gun as if it were loaded and ready to shoot, and never ever point them at people, even if I'm only pretending. When I'm done playing with my guns, I always make sure they are safe and clean. I put them in a safe place so my baby brother can't get them just like my dad does.

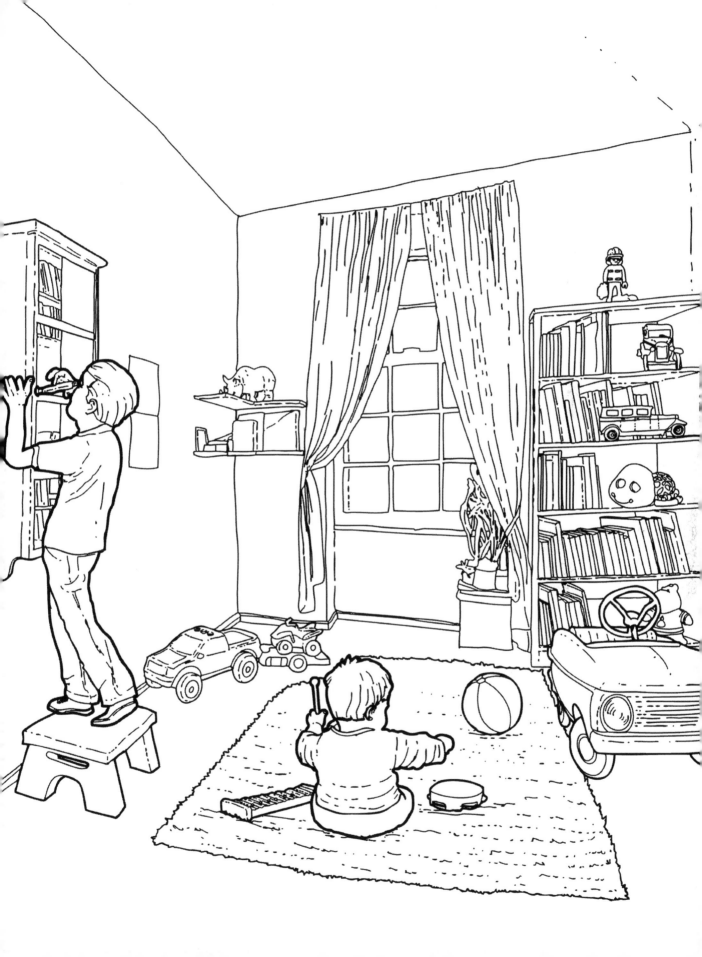

My dad has a big safe and it's bigger than me. His guns are always locked up in it. I know I'm NEVER EVER allowed to touch one without my dads help, and if I do see a gun somewhere it's not supposed to be, my dad taught me what to do.

1. STOP! Never ever touch it.
2. Tell any other kids around not to touch it.
3. Walk away from the area.
4. tell an adult right away.

I want to be safe, just like my dad.

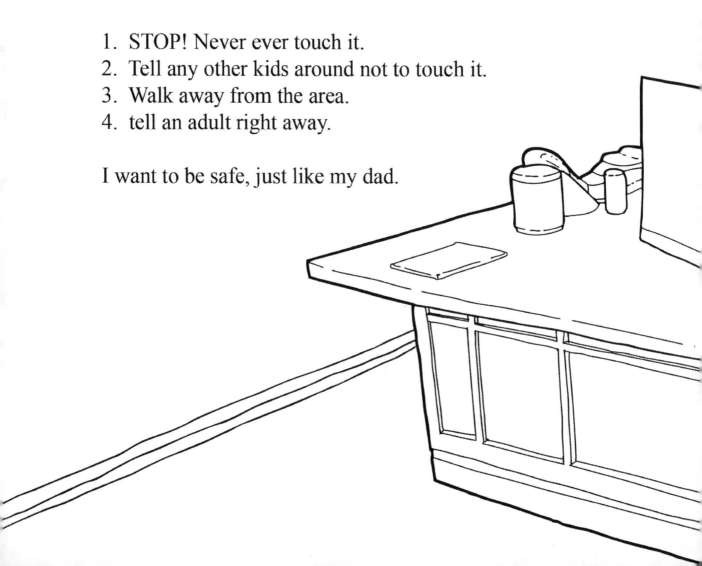

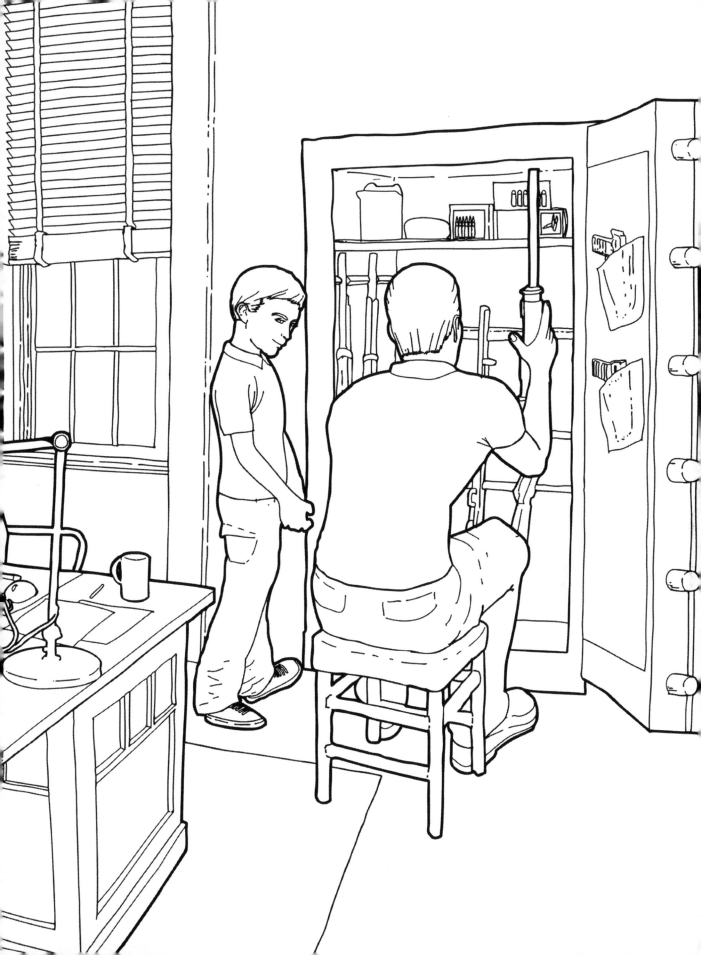

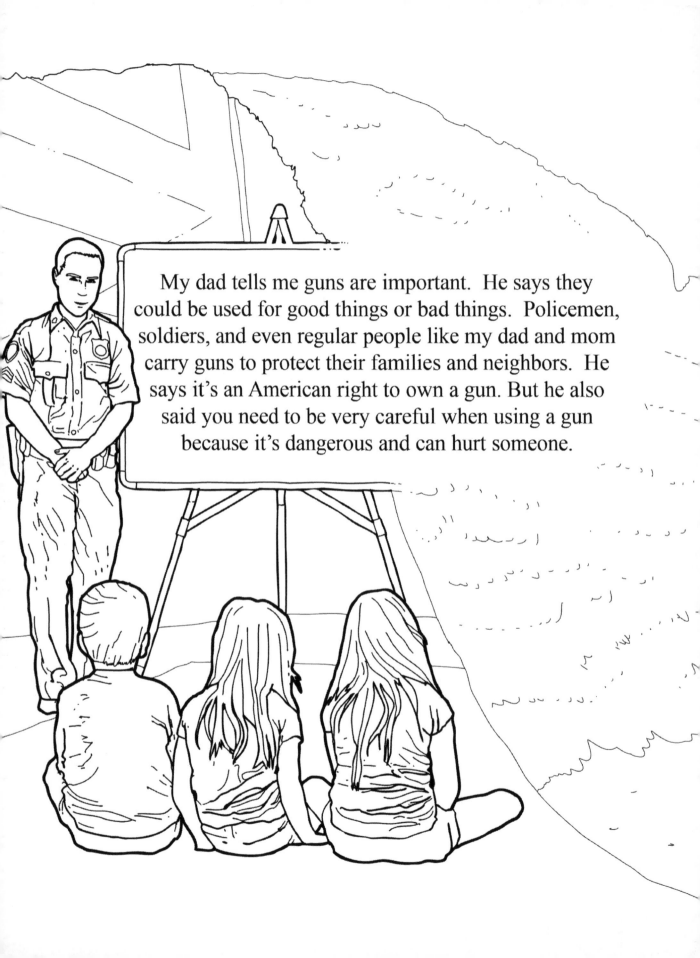

My dad tells me guns are important. He says they could be used for good things or bad things. Policemen, soldiers, and even regular people like my dad and mom carry guns to protect their families and neighbors. He says it's an American right to own a gun. But he also said you need to be very careful when using a gun because it's dangerous and can hurt someone.

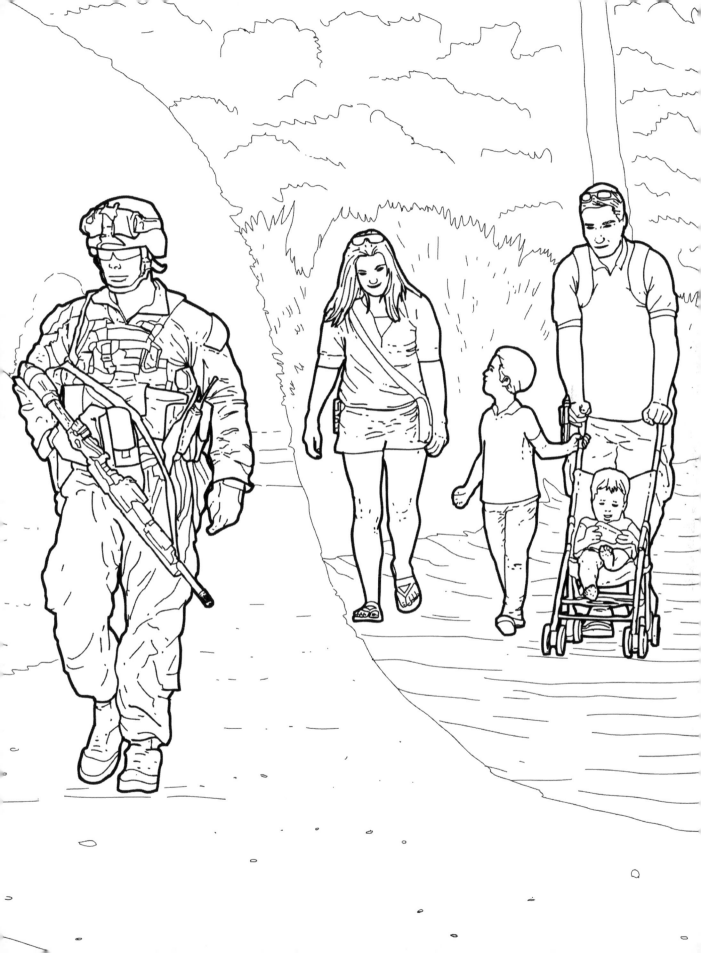

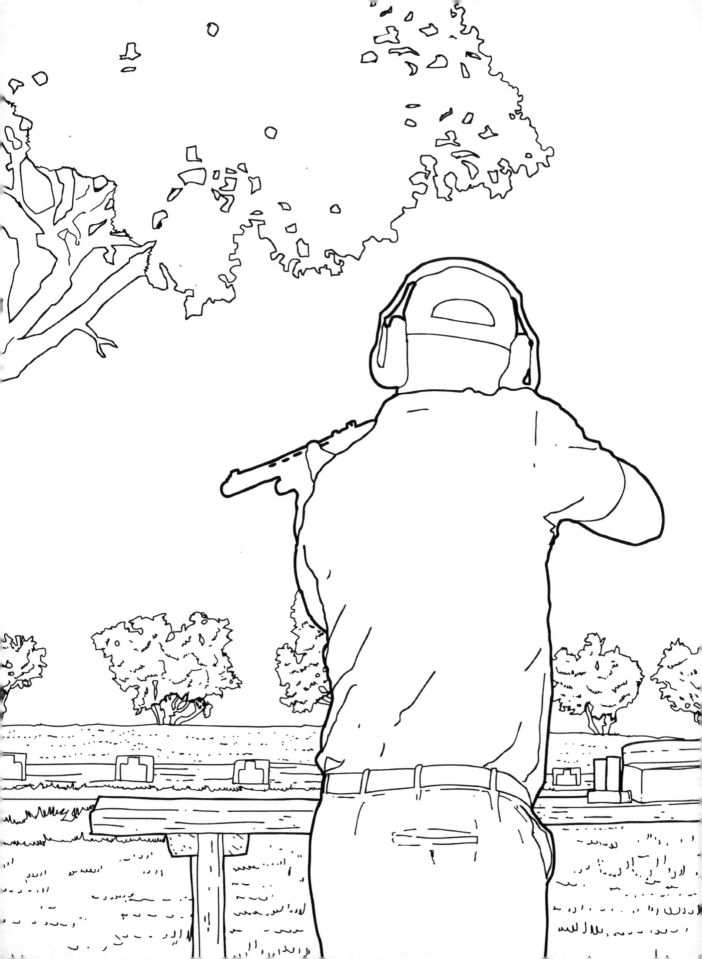

Sometimes my dad takes me to a gun range. It's a place where people can practice shooting their guns. Just like at home, there are special rules that you need to follow at a gun range.

A. Always wear ear and eye protection. You don't want to get hurt.

B. Treat all guns as if they are loaded.

C. Make sure the gun is always pointed down the range and away from people.

D. Always keep your finger away from the trigger until you are ready to shoot.

E. Before leaving make sure your gun is unloaded and the safety is on.

If you follow these rules, everyone will be safe.

When my dad comes home he again checks to make sure his guns have no bullets in them before he cleans them. He says "you need to be very careful so there are no accidents and no one gets hurt."

Before my dad puts his guns away in his safe, he always double-checks that the safety is on. The safety makes sure the gun can't fire or go off by accident. After he is done, I hold the safe door open so it won't close on my dad. He lets me check to make sure it's locked. We want to be as safe as possible.

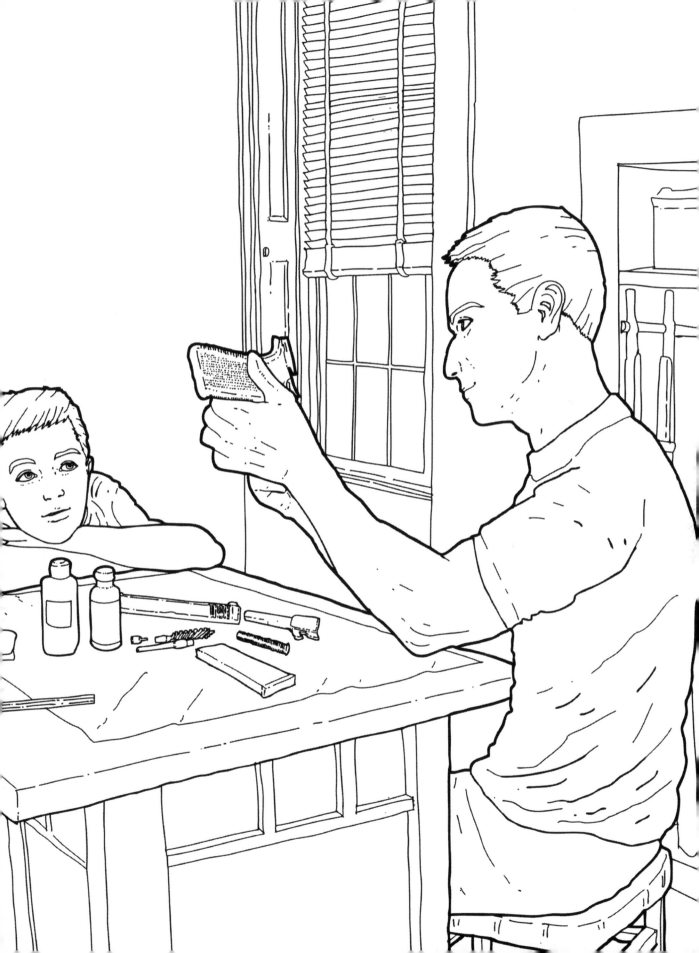

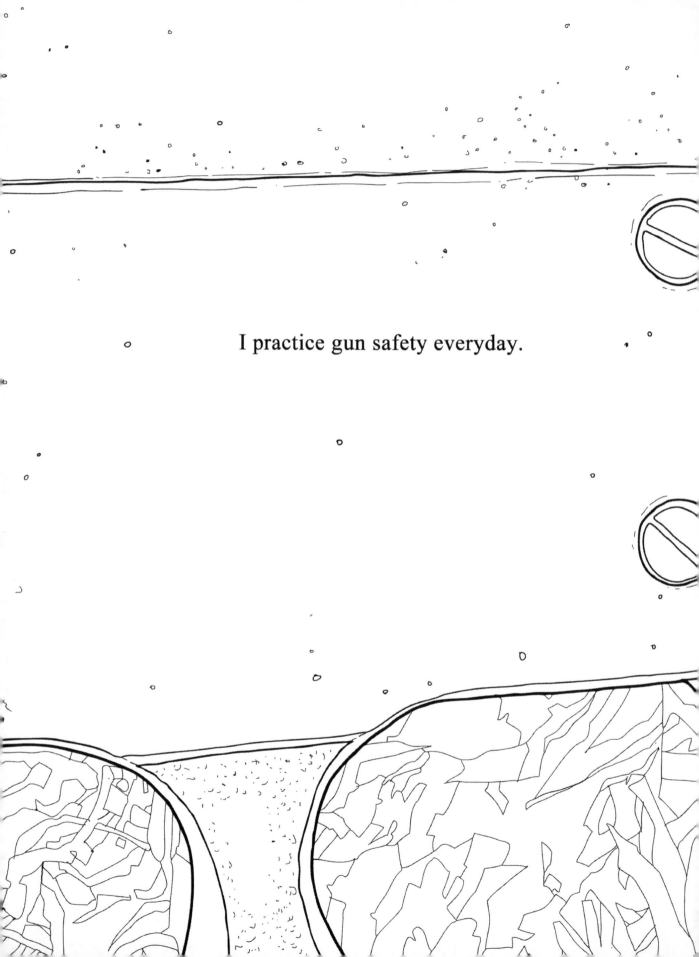

I practice gun safety everyday.

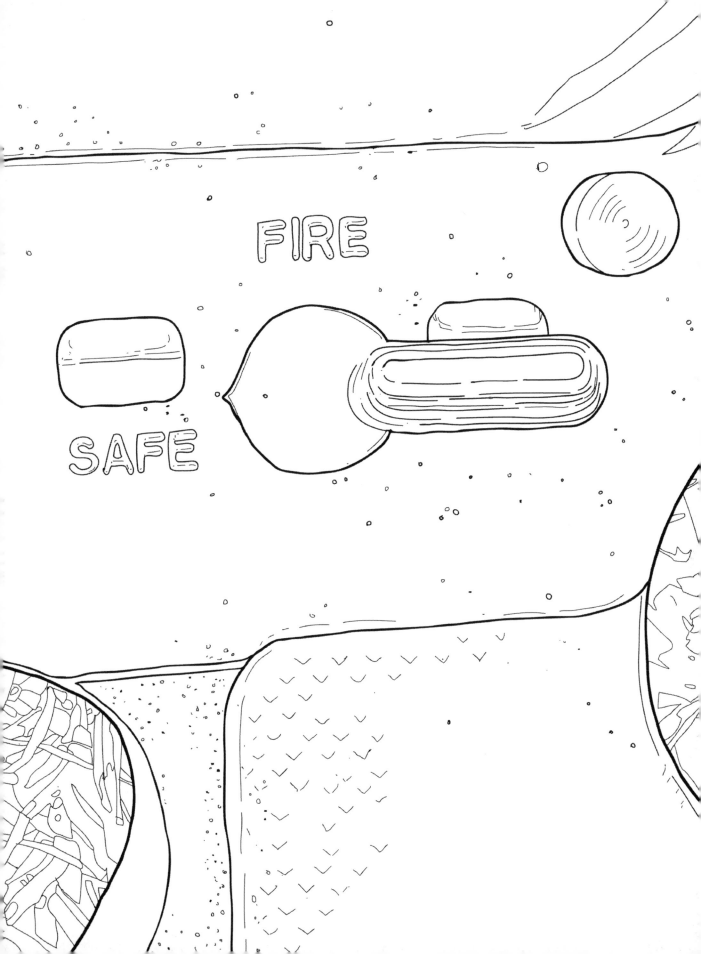

I know not to touch guns without permission.

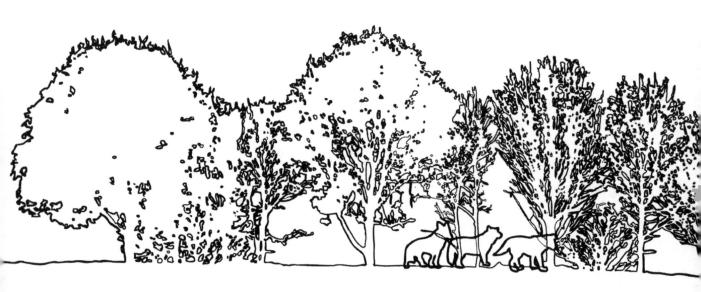

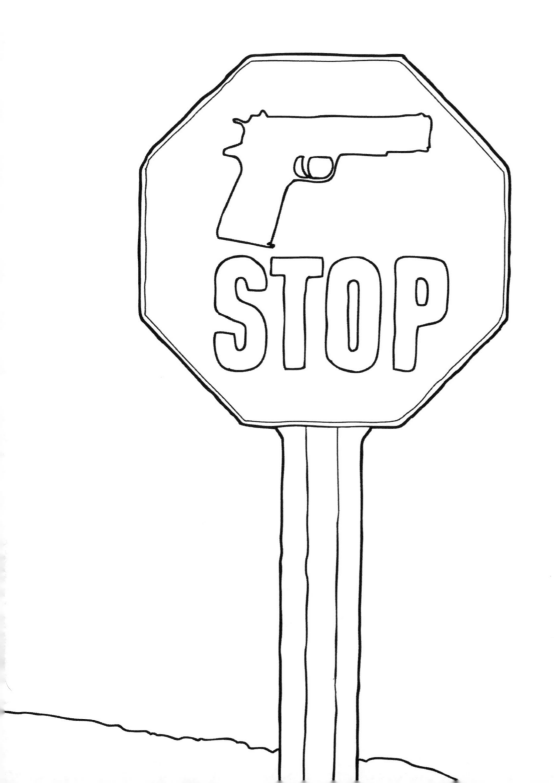

I know to tell an adult if I see a gun
somewhere it's not supposed to be.

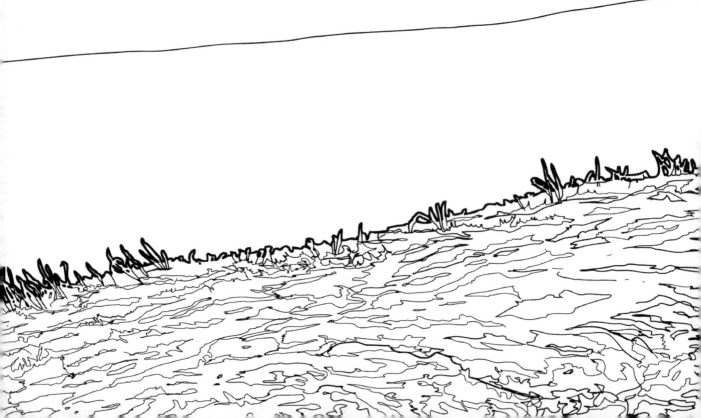

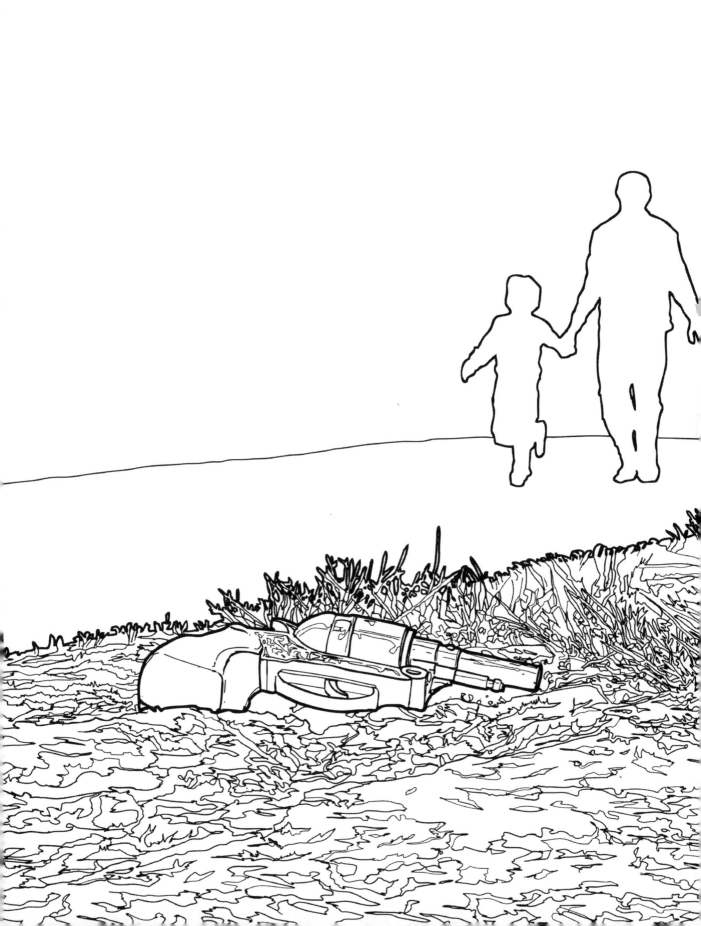

I never ever point my guns at anyone
even if I'm pretending.

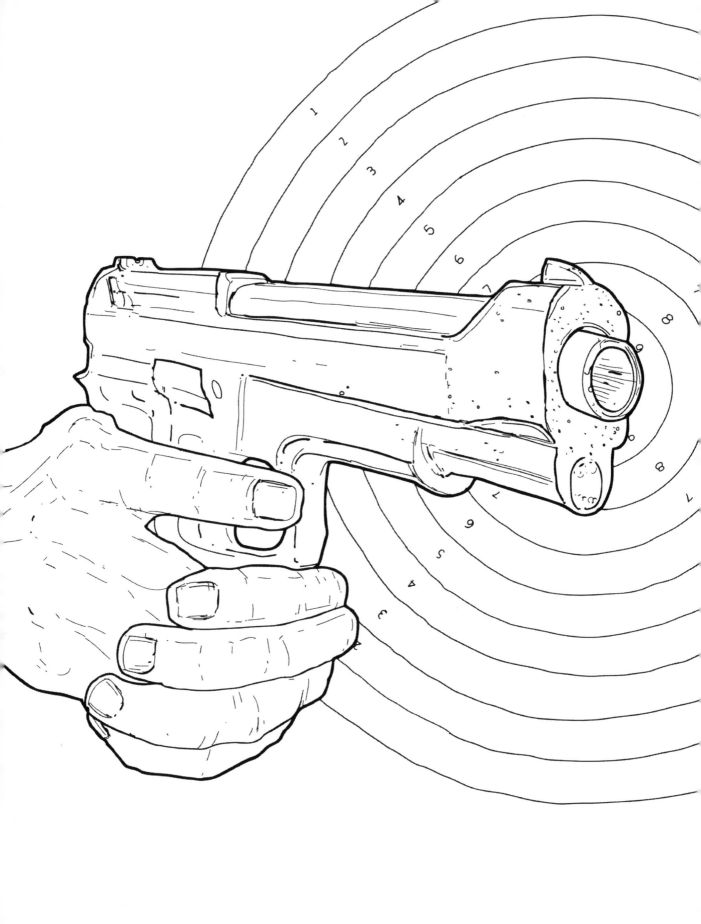

I put my guns away in a safe place
and make sure they are clean.

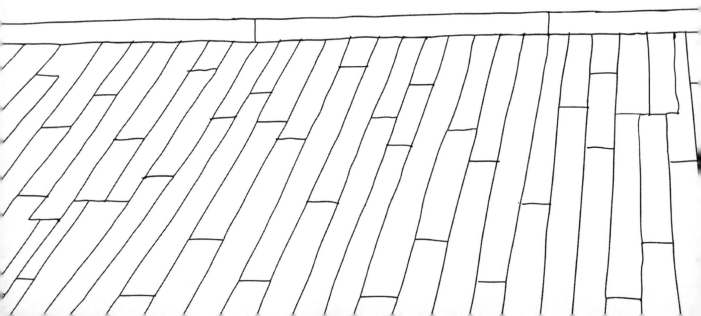

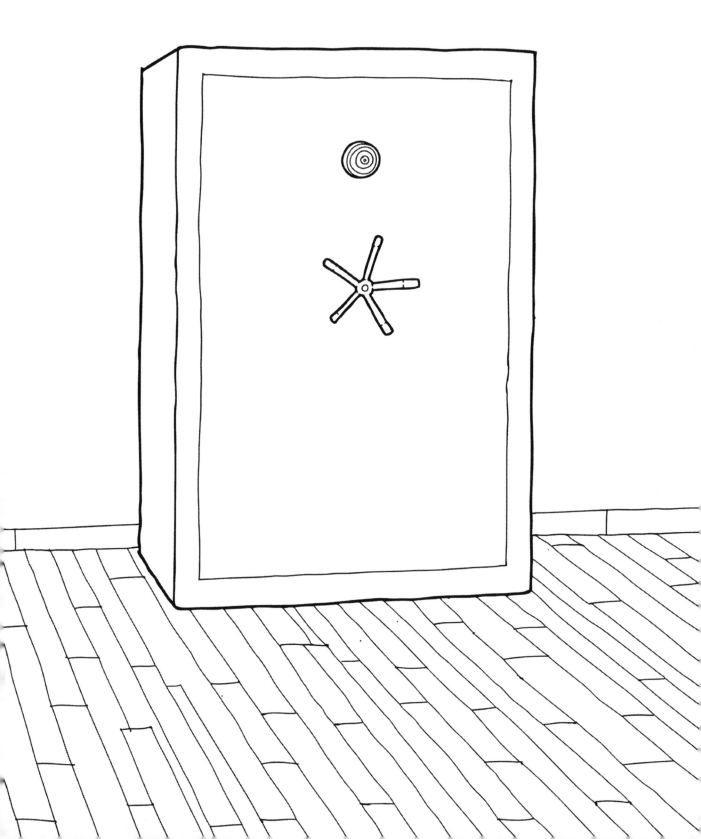

I treat all guns as if they are
ALWAYS loaded!

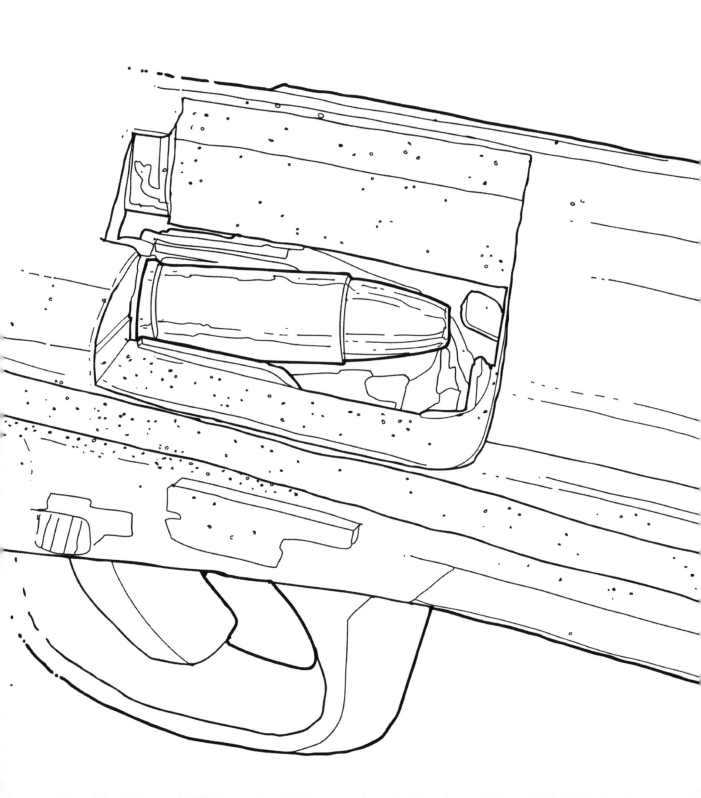

Never point your gun at anything
you are not willing to destroy!

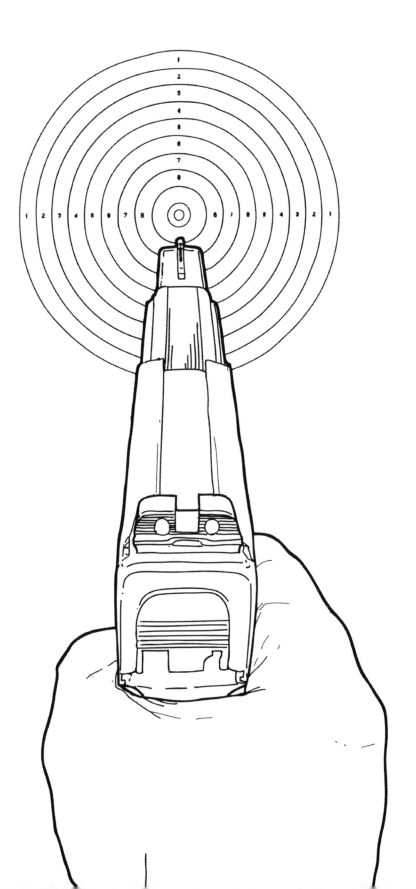

Keep your finger OFF the trigger and
OUTSIDE the trigger guard until you are
ready to shoot!

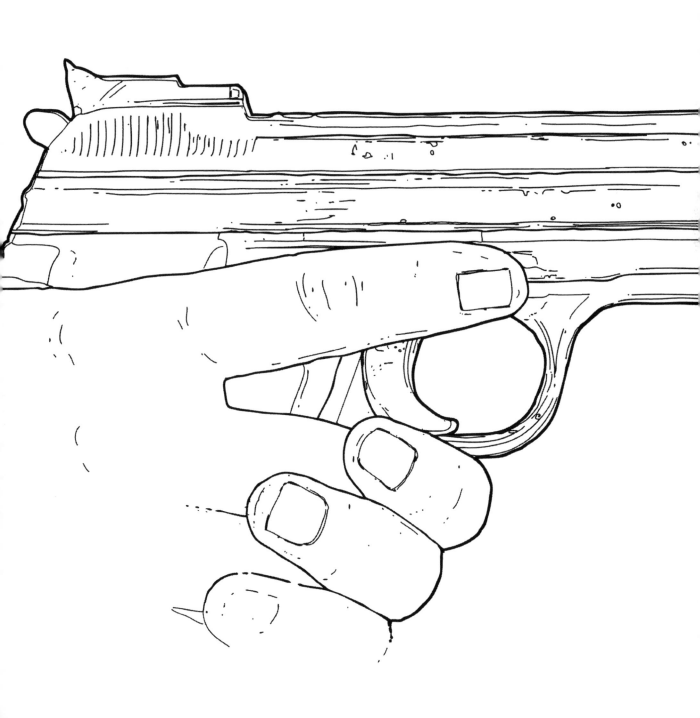

Know your target and what's
beyond it!

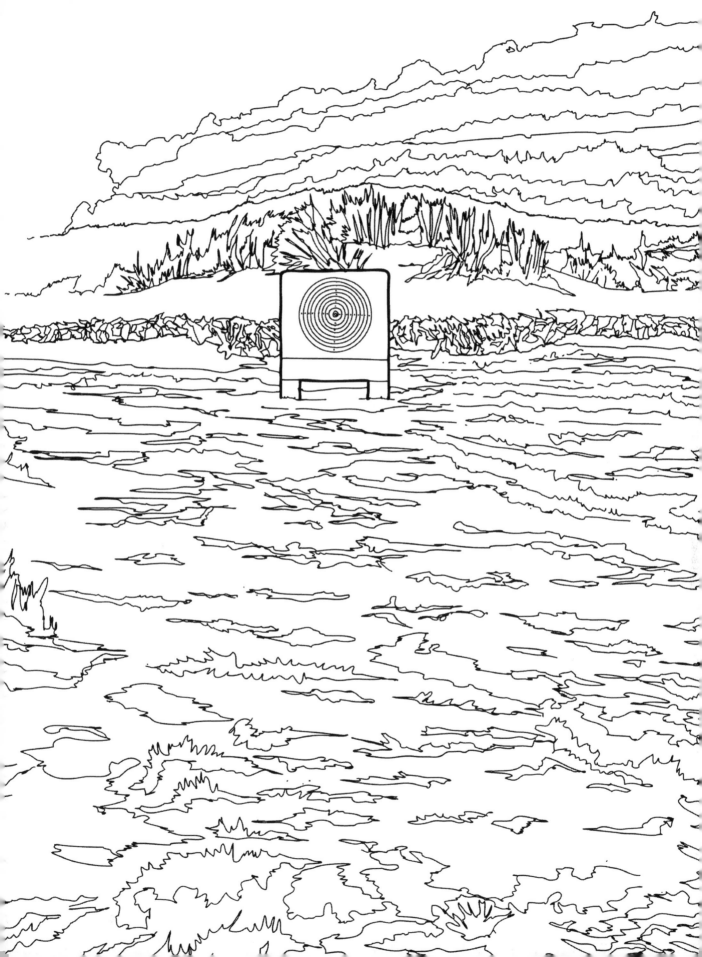

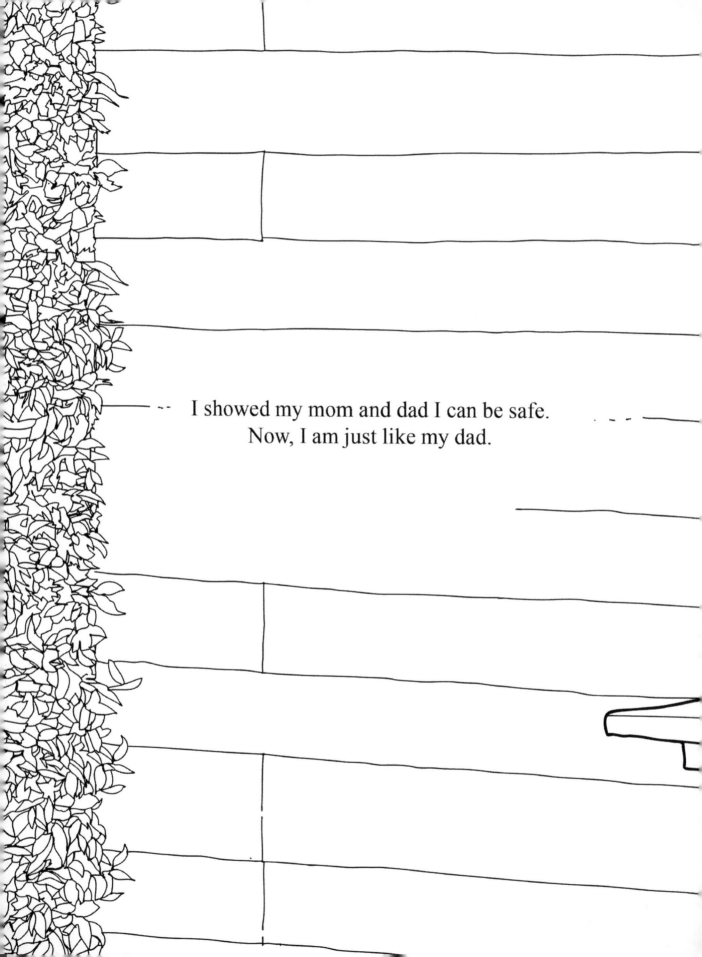

I showed my mom and dad I can be safe.
Now, I am just like my dad.

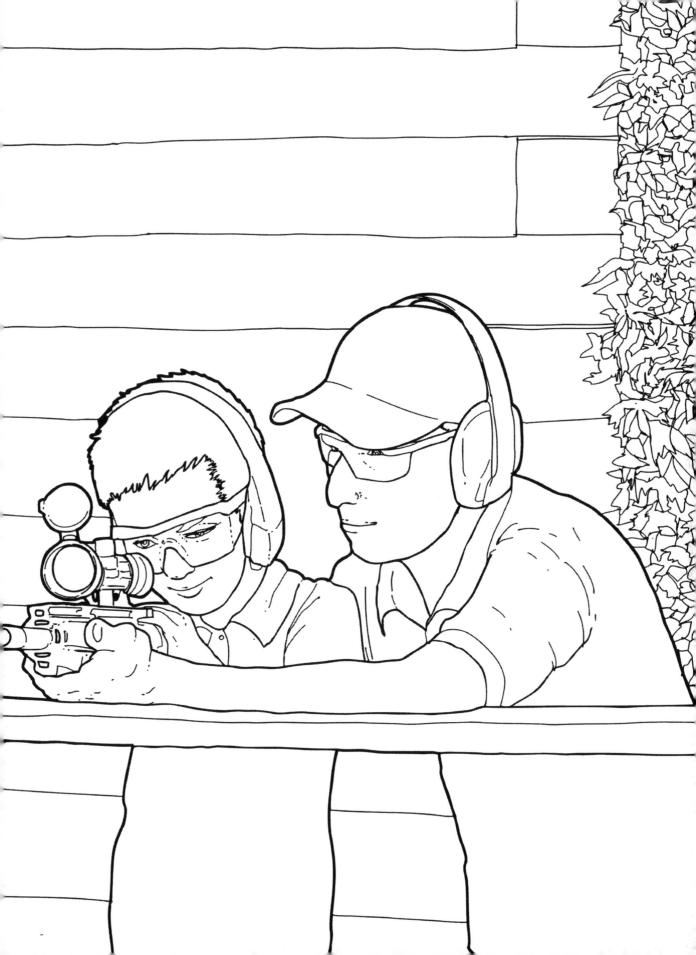

DO YOU KNOW THE RULES OF GUN SAFETY?

RULE#1: Treat all guns as if they are ALWAYS loaded!

RULE#2: Never point your gun at anything you are not willing to destroy!

RULE#3: Keep your finger OFF the trigger and OUTSIDE the trigger guard until you have made the decision to shoot!

RULE#4: Know your target and what's beyond it!

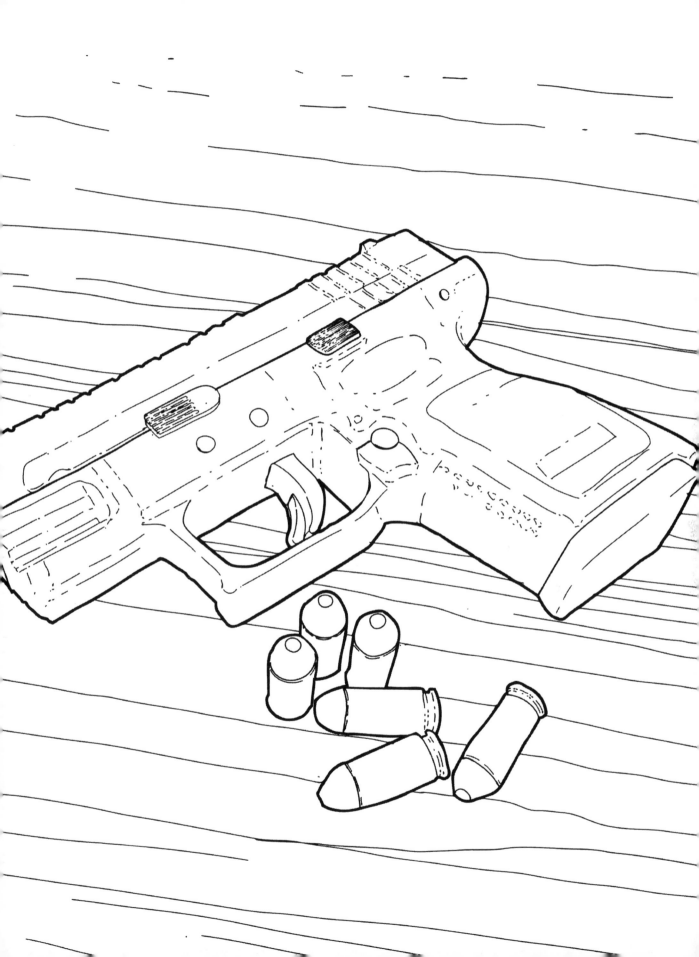

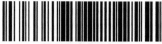

Manufactured by Amazon.com
Columbia, SC
06 April 2017